Table of Contents

Causes

Most cases of repeated (recurring) dyspepsia are due to one of the following:

Non-ulcer dyspepsia. This is sometimes called functional dyspepsia. It means that no known cause can be found for the symptoms.

Duodenal and stomach (gastric) ulcers. An ulcer occurs when the lining of the gut is damaged and the underlying tissue is exposed.

Duodenitis and gastritis (inflammation of the duodenum and/or stomach) - which may be mild, or more severe and may lead to an ulcer.

Acid reflux, oesophagitis and GORD. Acid reflux occurs when some acid leaks up (refluxes) into the oesophagus from the stomach.

Hiatus hernia. This occurs when the top part of the stomach pushes up into the lower chest through a defect in the diaphragm.

Medication. Some medicines may cause dyspepsia as a side-effect:

Anti-inflammatory medicines are the most common culprits. These are medicines that many people take for arthritis, muscular pains, sprains, period pains, etc. For example: aspirin, ibuprofen, and diclofenac - but there are others. Anti-inflammatory medicines sometimes affect the lining of the stomach and allow acid to cause inflammation and ulcers.

Various other medicines sometimes cause dyspepsia, or make dyspepsia worse. They include: digoxin, antibiotics, steroids, iron, calcium antagonists, nitrates and bisphosphonates.

H. pylori and dyspepsia

The germ (bacterium) H. pylori can infect the lining of the stomach and duodenum. It is one of the most common infections in the UK. More than a quarter of people in the UK become infected with H. pylori at some stage in their lives. Once you are infected, unless treated, the infection usually stays for the rest of your life.

Most people with H. pylori have no symptoms and do not know that they are infected. However, H. pylori is the most common cause of duodenal and stomach ulcers.

Symptoms

Dyspepsia is a term which includes a group of symptoms that come from a problem in your upper gut. The gut (gastrointestinal tract) is the tube that starts at the mouth and ends at the anus. The upper gut includes the oesophagus, stomach and duodenum. Various conditions cause dyspepsia. The main symptom is usually pain or discomfort in the upper tummy (abdomen).

Indigestion can feel like a stomach ache. You can have a range of symptoms including:

- pain, discomfort, or a burning feeling in your chest or stomach
- burping
- bloating
- gurgling stomach and/or gas
- acid reflux
- heartburn
- nausea and/or vomiting

Talk to your doctor if symptoms continue for more than two weeks. Seek medical care right away if your symptoms are severe, such as:

- shortness of breath
- trouble swallowing
- ongoing vomiting
- throwing up blood
- sudden pain in chest, arm, neck, or jaw
- cold sweats

- thick, black, or bloody stool

Diagnosis

A doctor will ask the person about:

- their symptoms
- their personal and family medical history
- any other health conditions and medications that they are taking
- their dietary habits

They may also examine the chest and stomach. This may involve pressing down on different parts of the abdomen to check for areas that may be sensitive, tender, or painful under pressure.

In some cases, a doctor may use the following tests to rule out an underlying health condition:

- Blood test: This can assess for anemia, liver problems, and other conditions.
- Tests for H. pylori infection: In addition to a blood test, these tests may include a urea breath test and a stool antigen test.
- Endoscopy: The doctor will use a long, thin tube with a camera to take images of the gastrointestinal tract. They may also take a tissue sample for a biopsy. This can help them diagnose an ulcer or a tumor.

Complications

In rare cases, severe and persistent indigestion can lead to complications. These include:

Esophageal stricture

Persistent exposure to stomach acid can cause scarring in the upper gastrointestinal tract. The tract can become narrow and constricted, causing difficulty with swallowing and chest pain. Surgery may be necessary to widen the esophagus.

Pyloric stenosis

In some cases, stomach acid can cause long-term irritation of the pylorus, the passage between the stomach and the small intestine. If the pylorus becomes scarred, it can narrow. If that happens, a person may not be able to digest food properly, and they may need surgery.

Peritonitis

Over time, stomach acid can cause the lining of the digestive system to break down, leading to an infection called peritonitis. Medication or surgery may be necessary.

How Can I Prevent Indigestion?

The best way to prevent indigestion is to avoid the foods and situations that seem to cause it. Keeping a food diary is helpful in identifying foods that cause indigestion. Here are some other suggestions:

- Eat small meals so the stomach does not have to work as hard or as long.
- Eat slowly.
- Avoid foods that contain high amounts of acids, such as citrus fruits and tomatoes.
- Reduce or avoid foods and beverages that contain caffeine.
- If stress is a trigger for your indigestion, learn new methods for managing stress, such as relaxation and biofeedback techniques.
- If you smoke, quit. Smoking can irritate the lining of the stomach.
- Cut back on alcohol consumption, because alcohol can also irritate the stomach lining.
- Avoid wearing tight-fitting garments, because they tend to compress the

stomach, which can cause its contents to enter the esophagus.

- Don't exercise with a full stomach. Rather, exercise before a meal or at least one hour after eating a meal.
- Don't lie down right after eating.
- Wait at least three hours after your last meal of the day before going to bed.
- Sleep with your head elevated (at least 6 inches) above your feet and use pillows to prop yourself up. This will help allow digestive juices to flow into the intestines rather than to the esophagus.

Treatments

Treatment for dyspepsia depends on the cause and severity. Often, treating an underlying condition or changing a person's medication will reduce dyspepsia.

Lifestyle treatments

For mild and infrequent symptoms, lifestyle changes may help. These include:

- avoiding or limiting the intake of trigger foods, such as fried foods, chocolate, onion, and garlic
- drinking water instead of soda
- limiting the intake of caffeine and alcohol
- eating smaller meals more often
- eating slowly

- maintaining a moderate weight
- avoiding tight-fitting clothing
- waiting 3 hours or more before going to bed
- raising the head of the bed
- avoiding or quitting smoking, if a smoker

Medications

For severe or frequent symptoms, a doctor may recommend medication. People should speak to their doctor about suitable options and possible side effects.

There are various medications and treatments available, depending on the cause of dyspepsia.

Medication options include:

Antacids

These counter the effects of stomach acid. Examples include Alka-Seltzer, Maalox, Rolaids, Riopan, and Mylanta. These are over-the-counter (OTC) medicines that do not need a prescription. A doctor will usually recommend an antacid medication as one of the first treatments for dyspepsia.

H-2-receptor antagonists

These reduce stomach acid levels and are more effective than antacids. Examples include Tagamet and Pepcid. Some are available OTC, while others are by prescription only. Some may carry a risk of adverse effects. A doctor can help a person choose a suitable option.

Proton pump inhibitors (PPIs)

PPIs reduce stomach acid and are stronger than H-2-receptor antagonists. Examples are Aciphex, Nexium, Prevacid, Prilosec, Protonix, and Zegerid.

Prokinetics

These can help boost the movement of food through the stomach. Examples include metoclopramide (Reglan). Side effects may include tiredness, depression, anxiety, and muscle spasms.

Antibiotics

If a Helicobacter pylori infection is causing peptic ulcers that result in indigestion, a doctor may prescribe an antibiotic. Side effects may include an upset stomach, diarrhea, and fungal infections.

Antidepressants

Sometimes, a problem with the central nervous system can lead to digestive problems. A low dose of an antidepressant may help resolve it.

Counseling

Chronic indigestion can affect a person's quality of life and overall well-being. Counseling may help some people manage these issues.

Options may include:

- cognitive behavioral therapy
- biofeedback

- hypnotherapy
- relaxation therapy

Drug interactions

If a person's medication appears to be a trigger for indigestion, a doctor may recommend adjusting the drug dose or type.

It is important to change medications only under the supervision of a doctor.

Dyspepsia diet

Dietary choices may help manage indigestion.

Tips include:

- following a healthful, balanced diet
- limiting the intake of spicy and fatty foods
- limiting caffeine and alcohol consumption
- drinking water instead of sodas
- avoiding acidic foods, such as tomatoes and oranges

Consuming four or five smaller meals per day instead of three larger ones can also help.

Dyspepsia recipes

ALKALINE SMOOTHIE

Ingredients

- 1 cup almond milk
- 1 cup watermelon cubed
- 5 strawberries frozen
- 1/2 small banana
- 1 handful spinach fresh
- 1 teaspoon chia seeds
- 1 cup ice

Instructions

- Place the ingredients into the blender as listed.
- Blend the smoothie until combined.

- To prevent a brown smoothie, mix the greens with the banana, chia seeds, half of the ice and half of the almond milk.
- Then blend the watermelon strawberries, almond milk, and ice together.
- Pour the smoothies into the same glass and enjoy.

Heartburn-Friendly Chicken Noodle Soup Recipe

Ingredients

- 1/2 tablespoon olive oil
- 1 cup trimmed and chopped celery
- 2 quarts water
- 2 cups peeled and chopped carrots

- 4 low-sodium chicken bouillon cubes
- 1/2 teaspoon thyme
- 1/2 teaspoon salt
- 3 ounces uncooked egg noodles
- 2 cups diced, cooked boneless skinless chicken breasts
- 2 cups frozen peas

Instructions

- Add 1/2 tablespoon olive oil to a large pot. Add 2 cup trimmed and chopped celery and sauté over a medium-high heat until translucent.   Add 2 quarts water, 2 cups peeled and chopped carrots, 4 low-fat chicken bouillon cubes, 1/2 teaspoon thyme, and 1/2 teaspoon salt. Bring to a boil.   Add 2 cups (3 ounces) large egg noodles to the boiling water. Stir. Return to a boil, reduce heat and cook for 8 minutes or until noodles are tender.

Add 2 cups diced, cooked boneless skinless chicken breast meat and 2 cups frozen peas. Return to a boil, reduce heat, cover and simmer over medium-low heat for 5 to 10 minutes.

Ginger Root Nature's Antacid

Ingredients

- Fresh ginger
- lemon
- water
- honey

Instructions

- Grate a small piece of Ginger (about the size of a nickel) into a mug
- Add the juice of 1/2 lemon.
- Fill the mug with boiling water.
- Stir in a teaspoon of honey. (raw and local, organic when possible)

Recipe Notes

- The even simpler version of this tea recipe...Slice 2 'coins' of ginger root and toss into your mug. I prefer to grate when time permits as a better digestive tea results..Your choice

TOASTED OATMEAL

INGREDIENTS

- 1 cup quick cook oatmeal (whole flake is also great, just double the cooking time)
- ½ cup water
- ½ cup milk
- pinch of salt

INSTRUCTIONS

- Add oatmeal to a saucepan. Over medium-high heat, stir it constantly for 2-3 minutes until toasted and a popcorn smell starts to appear. Don't over cook, and don't stop stirring or it will burn.

- Add all other ingredients. Bring to boil. Lower temperature and simmer for 3-4 minutes until thickened, stirring occasionally.
- Serve with your favourite toppings. I love yogurt, blueberries and pumpkin seeds.

Soothing Stomach Smoothie

Ingredients

- 1cupwaternut milk, or seed milk of choice
- iceoptional
- 1/2cucumber

- 1cupspinachkale, or chard (I recommend using pre-steamed smoothie pucks for reduced oxalates.)
- 1inchfresh ginger root
- juice of 1/2 lemon
- 1 tablespoondried chamomile

Instructions

- Add all ingredients to a blender.
- Blend on high until smooth.
- If using ice, add it last before blending.

Pineapple Ginger Tummy Soothing Smoothie

Ingredients

- 1 frozen banana

- 1 cup fresh pineapple
- 1/2 cup 2% or nonfat plain greek yogurt
- 1/4 cup unsweetened almond milk, plus more if necessary
- 1/2 teaspoons fresh grated ginger or 1/4 tsp ground ginger
- 1/2 teaspoons ground turmeric
- 2 teaspoons of chia seeds
- Optional: A few fresh mint leaves

Instructions

- Place all ingredients in a blender and mix until smooth. Pour into 2 glasses and enjoy immediately. Makes 2 smoothies.

Basic Millet Porridge

Ingredients

- 1/3 cup foxtail millets
- 4 cup water

Instructions

- Rince the millets with clean water.
- Cover the washed millets with 4 cups of water in a pot. Add more water if you prefer thinner porridge.
- Bring the pot to a boil and let it simmer with lid on for 30 mins. Stir once in a while to prevent the millets from sticking.

Notes

- The ratio of millets to water is based on the use of foxtail millets.
- If using other variety of millets, they may not make creamy and thick porridge.
- The calorie calculation is based on 1 serving.
- Make ahead tips: I love using my zojirushi rice cooker's porridge setting to make millets porridge. Set the ingredients and timer the night before and the porridge will be ready for breakfast when you wake up the next morning. Instant Pot is another good option to pre-program the porridge the night before.

Ginger Stomach Soother

Ingredients

- 1 cup raw sugar
- 1 cup water
- 1 pound fresh ginger root scraped mostly clean of its skin and roughly chopped then smacked with the side of a knife or meat tenderizer, divided

Instructions

- To Make the Ginger Stomach Soother Syrup:
- Stir the raw sugar and water together in a saucepan over medium high heat until the sugar is dissolved. Add about 2/3 of the ginger root and bring the mixture to a boil. Simmer for 5

minutes, then carefully add the remaining ginger root, remove the pan from the heat, cover and let stand for 30 minutes. Strain the syrup into a jar. Fix a tight fitting lid on the jar and store in the refrigerator.

- To Make a Ginger Stomach Soother Drink:
- Pour about 1/4 cup of the Ginger Stomach Soother over ice. Top off with fizzy or still water, as desired. Stir gently and sip to relieve an overindulged or sick stomach.

Healthy Gut Green Smoothie

Ingredients

- 10 –12 oz water or non dairy milk (coconut or almond or cashew)
- 1/2 small banana
- 2 tsp omega oil or mct oil
- 1 cup steamed spinach
- 1 scoop sprouted pea or brown rice protein
- 1/2 tbsp maple syrup
- dash of ginger root and cinnamon
- ice (optional)
- 1 scoop greens mix (supplement of choice) – Optional

Instructions

- Steam your spinach first. Just slightly in the microwave or stove top. This helps with digestions.
- Combine everything in blender and blend.
- Serve!

Turmeric & Ginger Anti-Inflammatory Dressing

Ingredients

- Juice from 2 large organic lemons
- 1" fresh ginger, skin removed
- 1 garlic clove
- 2 teaspoon ground turmeric
- 3 tablespoons extra virgin olive oil

- 1 tablespoon hemp seed oil
- 1 tablespoon apple cider vinegar
- 1 teaspoon raw honey (optional)
- ¼ teaspoon black pepper
- Himalayan salt to taste

Instructions

- Place all ingredients in a blender and mix until combined. Adjust seasoning as necessary.
- Pour over your favorite salad/mustard greens, protein, or roasted vegetables.

Black Bean Dip with Olives and Cilantro

Ingredients

- 1 can drained, rinsed black beans

- 3-4 Tablespoons soaked Cashews
- 2 Tablespoons olive oil
- 1 handful of cilantro
- 9-10 pitted black olives

Instructions

- Puree all ingredients in your food processor until smooth and creamy.
- Garnish with olives and cilantro.
- Enjoy with your favorite crisp or chip.

Banana Bread

Ingredients

- 3 very ripe bananas
- ½ cup honey

- 3 tablespoons expeller-pressed canola oil, plus a little more for oiling the loaf pan
- 1 teaspoon pure vanilla extract
- 1 ½ cups whole-wheat pastry flour
- 1 ½ teaspoons baking soda
- ¼ teaspoon salt
- ¾ cup chopped walnuts or pecans

Instructions

- Heat the oven to 350° F.
- Lightly oil a loaf pan.
- Mash the bananas and mix with the honey, canola oil and vanilla extract.
- Stir together the whole-wheat pastry flour, baking soda and salt.
- Add the nuts.
- Blend the two mixtures and spoon into a lightly oiled loaf pan.

- Bake for 40 minutes, or until center is set.

Papaya Salad

Ingredients

- 12 oz. Unripe green papaya (Peeled and cut in very fine matchsticks)
- 5 nos. Thai chili (fresh)
- 2 tbsp. Garlic (coarsely chopped)
- 3 Oz. Carrot (shredded)
- ¼ cup unsalted roasted peanuts (roughly crushed)
- ¼ cup Salad Tomato (cut in wedges)
- 1 tbsp. Palm or granulated Sugar
- 3 tbsp. Lime juice

- 3 tbsp. Fish sauce
- ½ cup Green cabbage

Instructions

- In a large mortar, pound the garlic and chilies roughly.
- Then add papaya and carrot, pound briefly or until they are broken down, but not completely mushy.
- Add the rest except peanuts and cabbage; continue pounding more gently so the liquids won't splash.
- Transfer to the serving plate, sprinkle with peanut.
- Serve accompanied by cabbage or any raw vegetables long beans, morning glory etc.

Cherries and Berries Smoothie

Ingredients

- 1 cup almond milk
- 1/2 cup frozen cherries
- 1/2 cup frozen strawberries
- 1 scoop vanilla plant-based protein of your choice
- juice of half a lemon
- 1/2 cup cooked white beans
- 2 tablespoons tahini

Instructions

- Simply combine all the ingredients in a high-speed blender until thick and creamy. You may adjust for your desired thickness by adding ice or removing liquid- the opposite is true if you prefer it thinner.

Peppermint Cinnamon Tea

Ingredients

- 1 tea bag, desired varieity
- 250 ml boiling water
- 2 ml Orange Naturals Peppermint Tincture (or substitute peppermint extract)
- 2 ml Orange Naturals Cinnamon Tincture (or substitute cinnamon extract)
- 1 tsp honey, to taste

Instructions

- Add tea bag to boiling water and let steep to desired strength.
- Add Orange Naturals Peppermint and Cinnamon Tinctures and stir briefly.
- Add honey to taste.

Notes

- Green tea is a great choice for this beverage for its extra antioxidants. Peppermint herbal tea provides additional anti-bloating benefits

Dairy Free Papaya Lassi

INGREDIENTS

- 1½ heaped cups ripe papaya
- ½ cup coconut yoghurt thick
- 2 tablespoons nut milk
- 2 tablespoons aloe vera juice or use extra nut milk
- Juice of 1 lime
- 2 teaspoons raw Manuka honey
- Few organic/spray-free rose petals
- ¼ teaspoon freshly ground cardamom
- Just a few chunks of ice
- Probiotic powder/capsule for extra good bacteria optional
- Crushed pistachios over the top

INSTRUCTIONS

- Blend all ingredients and serve.
- Sprinkle extra cardamom, rose petals and crushed pistachios if you have them, over the top to decorate.

Tomato-free pasta sauce

INGREDIENTS

- 3 medium celery stalks
- 3 medium carrots, peeled
- 2 medium zucchinis
- 1 medium beet
- 1/2 a small-medium turnip, peeled
- 2 cups of bone or vegetable broth (or more as needed)
- 7–10 fresh basil leaves

- 3–4 tbsp of grapeseed oil or extra virgin olive oil
- 1 tsp each of garlic powder
- 1/2 teaspoon of dried oregano
- 1 tsp of salt to add to sauce, plus a little more to season vegetables while cooking
- pepper to taste

INSTRUCTIONS

- Preheat oven to 400 degrees F.
- Prep vegetables: Peel the carrots and turnip. Cut the leafy tops close to the top of the beet, and trim the ends off of the zucchini, celery, carrots and turnip. Cut vegetables (except beet) into two-inch chunks. Since we will only be using half of the turnip in this recipe, you can either cook all of the

turnip or set the raw half that won't be used aside for use in other meals. Another option is doubling the recipe. Don't bother peeling the beet, as the skin is very tough to peel when raw. Peel it once it is cooked and slightly cooled.

- Spread the cut up zucchini, carrots, celery, turnip and out onto a large rimmed baking sheet lined with parchment paper. Drizzle with 2-3 tbsps of grapeseed or olive oil and sprinkle with desired amount of salt and pepper, then cover using parchment paper, tucking it snugly underneath.

- Wash the beet using a vegetable brush, then pat dry. Place in a baking dish lined with parchment paper and drizzle with 1 tbsp of olive oil. Cover using parchment paper, tucking the ends underneath.

- Place vegetables in preheated oven and cook until they are tender and can be easily pierced with a fork. Stir the carrots, zucchini, celery, and turnip occasionally while cooking.
- Once the beet is done cooking, let it cool slightly. Once cool, submerge it in a bowl of cold water and peel off the outer layer. Cut it in half and place that half in a high-speed blender or food processor. Feel free to add more if you want a deeper red color (keep in mind this will add a more earthy flavor to the sauce). Save the leftover beet for salads or other meals.
- Add the remaining cooked vegetables, broth, and fresh basil to the blender. Process until you have a smooth

consistency. Add the blended liquid to a saucepan along with the oregano, garlic powder, onion powder, salt, and pepper. Cook on medium-low for 4-5 minutes while stirring. Add more broth as needed for a thinner consistency.

- Remove from heat and serve with pasta or use as tomato/marinara sauce replacement.

Sweet and sour chicken

Ingredients

- 1/2 chicken, about 1 1/2 pounds
- 1 slice canned pineapple
- 1/4 cup rred wine vinegar
- 1/4 cup sugar

- 1/2 cup water
- 1 1/2 teaspoons dark soy sauce
- Dash of pepper
- Oil for deep-frying
- 1/4 teaspoon salt or to taste
- 1 clove crushed garlic
- 1/4 cup diced green bell pepper
- 2 teaspoons cornstarch mixed with 3 tablespoons water

Instructions

- Cut the chicken into 1-inch squares. Slice the pineapple into 1-inch pieces. In a small bowl combine the vinegar, sugar, water, soy sauce and pepper.
- Deep-fry the chicken in oil heated to 375 degrees for 5 minutes or until done. In a hot skillet or wok add 2 tablespoons of the oil and salt. Just

before the oil begins to smoke, add the garlic and stir until the garlic has become pungent. Add the vinegar mixture to the pan and bring to a boil. Add the carrots, bell pepper and pineapple. Add the cornstarch mixture. Stir until the sauce has thickned slightly. Pour the sauce over the chicken.

Reflux Friendly Banana Bread

Ingredients

- 1 1/2 c all purpose flour
- 1 /2 tsp baking soda
- 1 1/4 tsp baking powder
- 1/8 tsp salt
- 1/4 tsp cinnamon

- 1 c mashed banana
- 1/4 c vegetable oil
- 2 slightly beaten egg whites
- 1/4 c splenda
- non stick spray

Instructions

How to Make Reflux Friendly Banana Bread

- Blend together flour, baking powder, baking soda, cinnamon, and salt in a medium mixing bowl.
- •Blend together beaten egg whites, banana, sugar, and oil in a large mixing bowl.
- •Stir in flour mixture into the banana mixture, blending only until flour mixture is moistened.

- •Spray an 8x4x2-inch loaf pan with nonstick cooking spray. Spread batter in prepared pan.
- •Bake in a 350 degree F oven for 45 to 50 minutes or until a toothpick inserted near the center comes out clean.
- •Cool bread in the pan for approximately 10 minutes, then remove bread from pan and cool it thoroughly on a wire rack.

Lemon Balm Tea Recipe

Ingredients

- 3-5 fresh lemon balm leaves or 1 teaspoon dried organic lemon balm leaves

- 1 cup boiling water

Instructions

- Pour boiling water over the leaves, cover the cup with a plate, and let them steep for 5-10 minutes.
- Strain out the leaves and sweeten your herbal tea with honey, maple syrup,

Plant-Based Pea, Broccoli and Mint Soup

Ingredients

- 2 onion finely chopped
- 3 garlic cloves crushed then chopped
- 500 g frozen peas
- 1 head broccoli chopped

- 1 pint plant-based bouillon / stock
- 1 bunch fresh mint chopped. I used about 30 large leaves

Instructions

- Saute the onions for about five minutes until soft, then add the garlic and cook for another couple of minutes.
- Add the frozen pea, chopped broccoli, mint and stock then stir to combine the all together.
- Bring to a boil then turn down and simmer for 20 minutes until the broccoli is cooked through.
- Using either a hand blender, or counter top blender, blend the soup until smooth. Then ladle into warm bowls and serve with fresh crusty

wholemeal bread and a simple green salad.

COLOURFUL CHICKEN KALE SALAD

Ingredients

- 4 Medium Grilled or Stir-fried Chicken Breasts (1 per person)
- 1 Large Pomegranate - seeds removed
- 1 Cup of Brussels Sprouts
- 1 Head of Green Kale
- 1 Head of Purple Kale
- 1/2 Large Red Onion, sliced long
- 2 Green Onions, chopped
- 1/2 cup Coconut Smiles
- 1 cup of my Roasted Chickpeas
- 1 Large Avocado, cubed
- 1 Tablespoon Olive Oil

- 1/2 Tablespoon Grass-fed Butter
- 1 Tablespoon Fresh Tarragon, roughly chopped
- Dash of Himalayan Salt
- Dash of Black Pepper

For Dressing

- 6 tablespoons freshly squeezed lemon juice
- 1 clove garlic, minced
- 3 tablespoons extra-virgin olive oil
- 1 tablespoon Honey
- 1 teaspoon dried thyme
- 1 teaspoon Dijon mustard
- 1/4 teaspoon Himalayan salt
- 1/4 teaspoon black pepper
- 1/2 teaspoon finely grated lemon zest

Instructions

- Cook chicken, slice in long stripes and allow to cool.
- Make my Roasted Chick Pea recipe
- Wash, dry, and cut kale in bite size portions. Place in salad bowl and massage with olive oil and salt.
- Wash Brussels Sprouts and cut into halves, stir-fry on butter for 3-4 minutes and let cool.
- Slice onion into long thin pieces, salt all over (this is to ensure the taste is not too sharp).
- Place all ingredients in neat sections inside bowl, this allows all the colours to present beautifully.

Dressing Instructions

- Place lemon, dijon, honey, lemon zest, garlic, pepper, and salt into your blender.
- Slowly turn to high speed and blend for 30 seconds.
- Slowly add oils in a thin stream until emulsified.
- Reduce speed to medium and add thyme.
- Blend for an additional 30 seconds.

Raspberry Kombucha Smoothie

Ingredients

- For the Raspberry Layer
- 1 cup frozen raspberry (thawed)

- 1 tablespoon chia seeds
- For the Kombucha Layer
- 1/2 cup kombucha
- 1-1/2 cups oat milk
- 1 tablespoon rolled oats
- 1 tablespoon almond butter
- 1 banana (peeled, chopped)

Instructions

- Add the raspberries into a medium bowl and mash with a fork.
- Sprinkle in the chia seeds, then mix to incorporate.
- Set aside for 10 minutes to allow the chia seeds to absorb the liquid and turn the mixture into jelly.
- Meanwhile, prepare the kombucha smoothie by adding the ingredients

into a blender and processing to get a smooth, creamy liquid.

- Divide the raspberry chia jelly into two serving glasses. Then pour the kombucha smoothie evenly over the top.
- Mix and serve.

Digestive Salad

Ingredients

- 2 tbsp Botanica Daily Anti-Inflammatory Shot.
- 1/3 cup olive oil
- 2 cloves of garlic
- 2 tbsp apple cider vinegar
- 1/3 cup freshly squeezed orange juice
- 1 tbsp oregano

- 1/4 tsp black pepper
- pinch of salt
- 1/2 tbsp agave or maple syrup
- 3/4 cup uncooked quinoa
- 1 1/2 cups water
- 2 packed cups chopped kale
- 1/3 cup raw pumpkin seeds
- 3 medium oranges peeled and sliced
- 1 packed cup of grated carrots (roughly 2 large carrots)
- 1/3 cup green onions chopped

Instructions

- Place quinoa and water into a saucepan. Add a pinch of salt and pepper in and bring to boil.
- Cover with lid and cook for 18-20 mins. Until all the water is absorbed.

- Let cool for a few hours or put into the strainer and run under cold water to cool quickly.
- While quinoa is cooking make the dressing.
- Put olive oil, anti-inflammatory shot, apple cider vinegar, orange juice, oregano, black pepper, minced garlic, salt, and syrup into a food processor and pulse until blended. Or put into a jar with a lid and shake vigorously.
- The dressing should sit for 20 mins for the flavours to combine.
- Chop kale, carrots, green onion, and oranges.
- Toss in with quinoa into a large salad bowl and add in pumpkin seeds. Pour dressing over salad and toss.

- Serve in your favourite bowl. This salad is also great the next day as leftovers too!

Chinese Chicken and Rice Porridge (Congee)

INGREDIENTS

- 3 1/2 to 4-lb chicken, cut into serving pieces, including back and giblets (exclude liver)
- 10 cups water
- 3 tablespoons Chinese rice wine or medium-dry sherry
- 3 (1/4-inch-thick) slices fresh ginger
- 3 scallions, halved crosswise and smashed with flat side of a heavy knife
- 1/2 teaspoon salt

- 1 cup long-grain rice
- Accompaniment: fine julliene of fresh ginger, thinly sliced scallions, and Asian sesame oil
- N/A scallions
- N/A Asian sesame oil

Instructions

- Bring chicken and water to a boil in a 5-quart heavy pot, skimming froth. Add wine, ginger, scallions, and salt and cook at a bare simmer, uncovered, 20 minutes, or until breast meat is just cooked through. Trasfer 1 breast half with tongs to a bowl and continue to cook stock at a bare simmer, skimming froth as neccessary, 2 hours and 40 minutes. Meanwhile, cool chicken breast long enough to remove skin and bones, returning skin and bones to stock.

- Cool breast meat completely and tear into shreds. Chill shreds, covered, and bring to room temperature before serving.
- Pour stock through a large seive into a large bowl and discard solids. (you should have about 8 cups: if less, add water; if more, cook longer after adding rice.) Return stock to cleaned pot and add rice. Bring to a boil and stir. Reduce heat to low and simmer, covered until consistency of oatmeal, about 1 3/4 hours, stirring frequently during last 1/2 hour of cooking. (Congee will continue to thicken as it stands. thin with water if necessary.)
- Season congee with salt. Serve topped with chicken and accompaniments.